The Best Way to Get Rid of Varicose Veins Once and For All

Feel confident and sexy again

Table of Contents

Chapter 1:
Introduction

At first, I was not ready to share my secret about the varicose veins that I have. But I realized that I must share this because I am not the one who has it, and for sure, women have worse cases than mine. It is high time to share my story about my varicose veins and what I did to overcome my negative feelings.

I am a single mother with two beautiful children. I just had a birthday, and I turned 48, and although I am getting old, most of the people around me say I am aging gracefully. I work two shifts a day and work hard to raise my kids well. It was tough for me to work hard, and I think this is the second reason, aside from getting birth twice, why my varicose worsened.

I like this guy at work, his name is Jason, and I know the feeling is very mutual. He is adorable, he looks after me at work, and he is very interested in all the little things we talk about most of the time.

I still remember my first day in this company. Jason was one of the super lovely people by welcoming me and was always there to lend a helping hand if I ever lost. He was so friendly and very chatty. I did not expect that I would be very much interested in Him.

We mostly have coffee together, and as time goes, I can sense that we both have something in common. I told him about my children, and He was so open about His life story too.

At last, after several friendly chats and coy flirting, Jason finally asked me out for a dinner date. I took an hour early from work to look for the best outfit that my eyes could find in my closet. And finally, there it was, the perfect black sleeveless cotton dress. I was so excited that I wanted it to be perfect.

I bought it a month ago on sale without even thinking it was meant to but finally someone I like asked me out, and I am pleased, I know I will look good in it. It has been ages that I have not been on a date. I never really entertain any suitors, and for me, my children's welfare goes first.

So, I put my life on hold, and I never expected that I would still be interested in a guy. I want to look good because I like Jason, and I know He likes me too. I have the perfect dress, and I want this date to be perfect. Well, as the saying goes, "The first Impression lasts what happens next is up to you." I must nail it by looking extra hot.

I went home early that afternoon. Fix everything, and I am having a daydream about what will happen during dinner. The feeling is very overwhelming. I am so excited, and I am a little bit nervous.

I took a shower because I wanted to smell good all over. I put on the new favourite dress I bought, and I love how it feels and looks in my figure, one of my best assets aside from my long, lean legs and blonde hair.

I put some make-up on my face, and as I was combing my long blonde hair, I gazed at myself in the mirror. I look like a knockout, and I know that by the time Jason sees me, he will fall off his feet. I know that I am getting older, but I still have moved to make a man fall in love.

I was admiring how I looked, the dress fit perfectly, then suddenly there was the trace of my varicose veins and the new one peaking at me. I hurriedly grab the bottle of lotion and rub it in my legs, but there is no use.

I looked in my drawer at that old cream tube I bought way back and applied it to the areas in my legs that had varicose veins. And sadly, it has no use. I was a bit anxious at that moment because I had forgotten about it.

It has been long since I ignored it, for it didn't bother me that much. I often wear long pants or jeans at work, and I have not had a date in nearly two years now that I have never worn a dress for a very long time. I even forgot to buy a new tube cream or have it checked.

It is like nobody will look at it or even notice it until now that it's a reality check because I finally have a date and will have a good chance of being in a real relationship. I almost forgot how to take care of myself.

My life is routine, and I have no time to buy beauty products or deal with my varicose veins. I work two shifts with long hours, which is one reason I know why it does not look good now.

I have given birth to two nearly grown kids, and I am trying my very best to work hard as a single mom. I am always in a hurry. When I get home, I have to take care of my kid's needs, tuck them and make sure I am spending quality time with them, especially during my day off.

It was almost 8 pm, and I had to hurry because he was waiting for me at a fancy restaurant that I was dying to dine for a long time. Jason was extra nice remembering that I did mention to him about that restaurant, and I even told him that it was costly, yet he made a reservation and surprised me about it.

He was making a lot of effort, and I know He likes me. I took care of everything and ensured my children's needs were known before going out on my long-awaited date. I am crossing my fingers for this date. My goodness, I feel like I am 16 years old again.

On my way to the restaurant, all I think about is my stupid varicose veins. I am hoping he will never lay his eyes on it. I hurried back to the place, and then there he was; he looked fantastic and handsome.

He was holding a flower in his right hand, and he looked so adorable while waving his hand while I crossed the street. He was so lovely by reaching into my hand while I came across. He was even a gentleman by opening the door for me. I forgot all about this. It gives me an extra feeling that I haven't felt in a very long time.

My goodness, He looks so hot. He smells so good that as we walk to our table, I can still smell him in my hands. He smells earthy, woody as if He just went out of a shower.

I was beginning to enjoy the evening, The food, The ambiance, and The Man itself. As I was trying to have the most wonderful conversation, I was feeling a little bit confident. I suddenly reached my legs, and then there it was. I accidentally touched the area of my legs, and the horrible thought of my varicose veins hit me.

That is when I started to space out and lose interest. I cannot stop thinking about it. I cannot even hear Jason's voice and what he is talking about the whole time. I feel very conscious again.

The dinner ended, and I could not even imagine what happened for the last hours and minutes that we were having. I forgot some things that we talked about. And worst, I am not myself, and I have a dilemma about my varicose veins.

I was a disaster, especially by the time he took me in my car. I was so conscious that he might see my legs. He might notice my secret and that he will be turned off. Just because of it, I hurried back inside my car so that he didn't have a chance to bid a proper goodbye or even just give me a little kiss.

While driving my car, all I did was sigh and curse myself because I ruined a perfect first date with a guy I am so interested in.

I was not able to sleep that night and thought about what I had done that night. I am so angry with myself and these stupid varicose veins. I am rolling in and out of bed and just can't stop cursing myself and what I did.

The next day was my day off, and I was out doing some errands to buy some stuff at the grocery store nearby. As I was busy buying something from the grocery store, I bumped into an old friend of mine, and we decided to have a coffee afterward. We were catching up and talking about our past and how we were then. Young and fearless. She is still happily married and has kids whose age is like mine too.

I am so excited to tell her about my kids and my life at the moment. I brag about Jason and how I am so happy about it. I told her that I hadn't felt it for a long time. As I was telling her about my disaster date and that, I felt so bad because I ruined it just because I felt awkward about the idea of my varicose veins.

Gladly, she recommended a good doctor who treated her with her varicose veins too.

I was so glad that we bumped into each other, and this is not an end to my love life.

I finally gained the feeling of having another chance to get back to Jason for the bad ending in our date.

I hurried back home and called the number of the doctor, and luckily there was an opening late that afternoon. I went to see the doctor, and she told me that I am lucky to have it checked before it gets a more severe case of varicose veins. Then, she gave me some prescriptions and treatments. She gave me options in treatments as well as giving me products that were not that expensive.

The best thing is that you can choose whether to buy branded or generic products only. There are an array of variety and brands that you can choose from. I can say that I can be back on track again if only I have the discipline to follow my doctor's orders.

After two weeks of using the prescribed products, I find it amazing because I can see the results already. My affected area is beginning to glow. The veins are not that bad like it was.

It gives me an urgent feeling to continue using it and to the extent that I put it in my daily activities to not forget.

I've been taking my medications religiously, and I am getting more promising results.

I also eat rich in fibre and somehow find time to do some exercises at least once a week.

Honestly, I have realized that I am not only doing this for Jason, but I am doing it for myself and my children. I finally have the time to love myself and take care of myself, which I haven't done in a very long time.

I feel healthy. I feel good as well; I feel young and attractive again. I find it hard to believe, but It gives a certain glow to my face that gives me extra self-confidence. And most people notice it and keep on asking me, "What's with you lately"?

I never hesitated. I said yes. He was extra sweet to me for the past couple of days, always asking about the kids and all, now I know that He wanted to meet them.

I was so excited that I told my kids over dinner. I don't know why I am not worried about what my kids will say, maybe because I know them too well and that they are ok with the idea of me dating. Gladly, they said yes.

I was confident that I was not even worried about what to wear or maybe to think that I could wear anything. The day has come, and to my delight, my kids and Jason made the best impression with one another.

We were having a good time, and suddenly He put his arms around me and said: "You look gorgeous; you took my breath away." I was wearing a mini dress, and I could see a slight trace of my varicose veins, but it did not look the same as before. I can say that the improvement is very impressive.

The day ended with my kids very happy and the fulfilment that I gave Jason a great time. I made new good memories with Him and made a good impression, unlike the disaster date.

As we said our goodbyes, he grabbed me by the waist and gave me the most beautiful, passionate first kiss. I can feel the warmth in his kiss that I almost want more. It was the best date I have ever been to, watching my kid's happy spending day with the man I like. Well, the next thing is history, you know.

I am having the best time of my life, and I thank my friend for giving me the answers to my worries by showing me that excellent doctor who prescribed me medication and telling me what's the best thing to do about my varicose veins.

Up to this day, I still take care of myself and prevent my varicose from growing again.

I am combining over-the-counter creams and home remedies and, of course, keep checking my doctor to make sure I am doing the right thing.

For me, Prevention is better than cure. So, there is my story that I want to share with all the ladies who suffer and have a problem like mine. It is not the end of the world. All you have to do is ask for professional help or be informed and be well aware.

Don't be afraid to find a way to solve your problems. Don't hesitate and be ashamed to ask for help. Try to love yourself by taking care of it so that you can live a happy life.

Chapter 2:
Finding the Perfect Way to Get Rid of Varicose Veins

Dealing with a problem with varicose veins is rather painful, uncomfortable, and some lead to low self-esteem. I even took it as a severe problem. It gives us the feeling of being unattractive, and we feel conscious about it. Some people who have serious issues must undergo surgery to correct them.

Most women have it by giving birth, and some develop it by working non-stop especially if your line of work requires much standing. But as we all know, varicose can happen in any part of our body, but the common area is the legs.

They are considered a severe medical condition, but they can be very uncomfortable and lead to more severe problems. Here are some home and everyday tips on how to deal with varicose veins.

1. Consult the best Doctor you can find. Look online or ask a friend to help you find a good doctor for that. They will conduct some tests, and they will give you prescription medicine.
2. Never miss a prescribed medicine that the Doctor gave you. She will provide you with time to find out if the medication she gave you works, and she will have you a follow-up check-up.
3. Do a Self-Care ritual such as keeping your body moving, losing excess weight, wearing comfortable and loose clothes, elevating your legs, and avoiding long periods of standing or sitting. It can help you ease some discomfort

and to prevent your varicose veins from getting worse.

4. Buy and Use Compression Stockings. It can help your muscles move blood more, and they steadily squeeze your leg muscles, supporting your veins and muscles. You can buy it in many drugstores, department stores, or you can buy it online.

5. If your case is a little bit severe, follow your doctor's order and treatments or seek another Doctor's opinion, or you can undergo some surgery treatments. He knows best and what is best for you.

Chapter 3:
Home Remedies You Can Use to Relieve Varicose Veins Pain

Here are some home tips on how to ease the pain you experience from your varicose veins.

1. Exercising. You can try different kinds of exercise like walking, swimming, or biking.
    These types of exercises will help your veins move blood with compression.
2. Watching your weight. Always watch what you eat. Have a healthy diet and always be watchful of your daily food intake. Try to monitor your weight every day.
3. Eating a high fibre, low salt diet. High fibre food and diet includes whole grains, popcorn, potatoes, and fruits like avocado, berries, apples, pears. It is also a low salt food. You have to have a portion of healthy food and a healthy lifestyle.
4. While taking a nap, elevate your legs or put on a pillow that works in your comfort. Elevating your legs if you are resting gives your legs time to relax, and it will normalize the blood in your legs. Do it at least once or twice a day.
5. Changing your sitting or standing position regularly. It can help blood flow in your legs. You can prop up your legs when sitting, avoid crossing your legs at the knees when sitting. Don't stand too long; always sit and rest awhile.
6. Avoid wearing high heels or tight shoes. High heels and closed shoes are not suitable for varicose veins. It puts pressure on your legs which is not ideal for you.

Chapter 4:
What are the Symptoms of Varicose Veins

The common symptoms and causes of varicose veins are different for different kinds of women. I don't feel any pain, unlike other women. I feel a little discomfort, but it is tolerable for me.

Spider veins are similar to varicose veins; they are a little smaller. Spider veins are found closer to the skin's surface and are often red or blue. They occur on the legs but can also be found on the face. These veins can be in different sizes, but all have one thing in common, they often look like a spider web.

Here are some common symptoms that are known to all:

1) Veins turning dark purple or blue. These symptoms are most common on your legs.
2) veins that appear twisted and bulging; they are often like cords on your legs. This kind of varicose vein is the most painful one.
3) An achy or uncomfortable feeling in your legs.
4) Burning, throbbing, muscle cramping, swelling, and a tingling sensation in your lower legs.
5) Worsened pain after sitting or standing for a long time.
6) Itching around one or more of the veins.
7) Skin discoloration around varicose veins.

Chapter 5:
Causes of Varicose Veins

Most women who are aging and have given birth to one or more kids are prone to varicose. Being female, having a hormonal imbalance is a big deal.

Aside from that, here are the other causes of varicose veins.

1) Getting older - is an issue when it comes to varicose veins. The more you age, the more you are prone to it.

2) Pregnant- having kids is one of the leading causes of varicose veins. As we get pregnant, our hormones change, and we gain weight, so is it possible for varicose veins to develop.

3) Obesity- is most common in women. We have kids; we are getting older; we don't watch what we eat. We let ourselves go because we find comfort in junk foods and unhealthy diets.

4) Standing for extended periods- most women who have a job that requires a lot of standing are very prone to it. Having jobs like mine, double shifts, and working long hours every day are most likely to develop.

5) Unhealthy lifestyles like smoking - although smoking does not necessarily cause varicose veins, you are more likely to have them if you do smoke. Varicose veins also raise your risk for a condition called deep-vein thrombosis, which can lead to the development of life-threatening blood clots.

6) Genetics- just like many gene disorders, varicose veins are, in fact, hereditary. Your risk of developing varicose veins increases if a close family member has the condition.

7) Being inactive- women who don't exercise and don't do much often tend to develop varicose veins.

I am one of those women. I even let myself work as hard as I could, standing for an extended period just to earn for my children.

As I get older, I have noticed that although I am not like other women who experience a lot of pain, I still developed more varicose veins due to my line of work. I also don't have time to exercise and mostly find comfort by not eating right.

Here are some essential things you should know that can lead to causes of varicose veins and can lead to weak or damaged valves.

- Arteries that carry blood from your heart to the rest of the tissues that make up your body struggle to circulate normally.
- These veins should return blood from your body to your heart and recirculate the blood, but it cannot recirculate due to the varicose veins, leading to damaged valves.
- Muscle contractions in your lower legs act as pumps, and elastic vein walls help blood return to your heart.
- All the tiny valves open as blood flows toward your heart, then close to stop blood from flowing backward. If blood cannot flow backward, it means that the valves are weak and damaged.
- It can cause veins to stretch or twist.

Chapter 6:
Complications of Varicose Veins

Some women have severe cases of varicose veins. Most experience a lot of pain, especially if their Veins are somewhat more prominent, and it develops an uneasiness or discomfort that varicose veins can't easily ignore into your life for long periods at all.

Certain complications also develop, such as;

1) Ulcers- Deciding against varicose veins treatment may lead to chronic skin inflammation and surrounding tissue. Over time the skin breaks down, and forms an open wound, called an ulcer. Painful ulcers may form on the skin near varicose veins, particularly near the ankles.
2) Blood clots- Occasionally, veins deep within the legs become enlarged. You may experience bleeding or weeping in the ulcer, and it may become infected.
3) Bleeding may occur. - Veins very close to the skin may burst, and it can cause bleeding.

Most untreated varicose can cause moderate to severe complications. It can result in more severe complications. However, it is a low, potentially life-threatening condition known as "deep vein thrombosis (DVT). A blood clot forms in the lower leg or thigh, resulting in severe blockage of the veins and arteries.

Most women often ignore varicose veins and choose not to be treated. It can raise specific issues like this. Most of us don't find the time or are too lazy or too busy. We can give several reasons, and at the end, we are the one who suffers and feel anxious about it. We must not neglect this kind of issue.

We owe ourselves to be healthy and on the go. It doesn't mean that we have to let ourselves go as we get older. We ought to take care of ourselves and have a healthy lifestyle.

Chapter 7:
Effects of Varicose Veins

Men and women over 40 can have varicose veins. Most women between the age of 40 to 80 years old have it. Female hormones are thought to play a role in this. We are at most risk of having it.

Effects can be a little bit annoying. Based on my own experience, I can feel a little less pain and discomfort. I sometimes forget I have it because I don't usually wear dresses that show it off. Still, some women, especially working in the office, typically wear corporate attire, including skirts. So, they find it odd, and most of them don't like the way it looks.

First of all, they must wear stockings, and some women don't like wearing them. On the other hand, I don't wear dresses now, and I just realized it when I ended up on a date.

Here are some common effects on women who have varicose veins:

1) Pain or aching in parts where they have it. - We feel pain, and most of the time, it gives a heavy feeling. Some over-the-counter medicine gives a short remedy for it. The pain usually came back, and at that time, we mostly felt uncomfortable. We must seek professional help for this, and sometimes it costs a lot of money.

2) Swollen feet and ankles- Swollen is a word you can connect to discomfort and pain. If something is swelling, it hurts. Some can't walk or have a hard time walking. It is not a great feeling, and it can cause you a lot of distress because you cannot do anything.

3) Burning or throbbing in your legs- Hot and burning

sensations may occur in the affected area of your legs or any parts of your body. It usually happens if the damaged veins allow blood to pool within your legs.

4) Muscle cramps in your legs, particularly at night-varicose veins and underlying venous insufficiency are common causes of night cramps. It is mostly at night because we don't have any activity. The most commonly affected are the upper legs. It often wakes us up in our sleep, and it is sometimes hard to move, so it is very discomforting.

5) Dry, itchy and thin skin over the affected vein- varicose veins itch because of a condition called venous stasis dermatitis. The skin over the veins becomes red and itchy due to the blood that builds up and damages the vessels. It eventually leaks out into the skin.

Some effects of varicose veins are long-term. Factors that increase the development of varicose veins can be crucial. Issues such as Sex, age, and genetics are the most common factors for this. But we can still work out the effects if we treat it or let it be treated.

Finding professional treatments and using products that you can buy over the counter or home remedies can reduce its development or cure. In that way, we will not worry about the effects on us.

Chapter 8:
How to Prevent Varicose Veins

Preventing varicose veins is better than curing them. If you are a woman of a specific age and have signs and symptoms of developing varicose, you may experience a minimal or worst feeling.

Hormonal imbalances and being pregnant is a most common trace of having this. Lifestyles are also one of the significant contributors to it. As the saying goes, prevention is better than cure. So, it is like the same in-home remedies on how to ease what you are feeling.

Here are some practical tips on preventing varicose veins:

1) Get moving. Exercising and performing specific activities like swimming and walking are only examples of getting on the move. It will help you not to develop varicose and get fit.
2) You have to watch your weight and your diet. The more fit and slim you are, the healthier. Shedding excess pounds takes unnecessary pressure on your veins. Eating food with low salt and more fibre is the best way of losing weight. Be watchful of your diet to avoid developing varicose veins.
3) Watch what you wear on your feet. Avoid wearing high heels and tight shoes. Through your legs will be out of stress and pressure.
4) Avoid standing or sitting still for an extended time. If you are sitting, avoid crossing your legs. Make sure that if you stand, always take time to sit down and rest your legs.
5) Elevate your legs. Have this habit at least 2 to 3 times a

day. It is the best way of relaxing your legs. It relieves pressure and makes your blood flow well.

Some factors may increase the risk of developing varicose veins. Aging causes wear and tear on valves in your veins that help you regulate blood flow. It means that the more you age, the more you are prone to it.

If most women are well informed about this, they can be aware that the earlier you take care of yourself and get yourself treated, the better. Preventing varicose veins is much better than curing them.

Chapter 9:
Things to Know Before Any Varicose Vein Procedure

Some people who have severe cases of varicose veins must undergo surgical treatments. Some must receive laser treatments that health professionals can only administer. There are some risks of laser treatment. It is essential to be aware and well-informed. To achieve optimal results before and after your vein procedure, Have a heart-to-heart talk with your doctor. I suggest you follow your physician's orders.

Here are the pre- and post-common things you should know:

Pre-Treatment Instructions;

- Your doctor may advise you to stop taking medications like aspirin or anti-inflammatory drugs before any procedures. It may be prescribed, or any over-the-counter drugs for it may cause heavy bleeding or any complications.
- Avoid taking beverages that are caffeinated before your procedures. But, make sure you are well hydrated.
- Make sure to have eaten your breakfast. Never take the procedure with an empty stomach.
- Wear loose clothing and bring your compression stocking on the day of your procedure. You might be needing those after your surgery.
- Make sure you arrange a ride home or, better yet, bring some company with you because you are not allowed to drive after your procedure.

Post Treatment Instructions;

- Rest. You need to take it easy for 1 to 2 weeks. This treatment will prevent you from avoiding bruising, bleeding, and pain. Make sure to sleep and eat well for a fast recovery.
- Don't take a bath or take a shower for at least two days. You can have a sponge bath, but make sure that the affected areas won't get wet, or better yet, ask your doctor how many days or weeks not to get your incision from being wet.
- Decline from having strenuous activities. Avoid doing heavy exercises like aerobics, extreme walking, or bicycling. Take it slowly for a while.
- Eat more fibre-rich food. Surgery can affect your bowel movement; it is better to have this diet so that your bowel will return to normal sooner.
- Ask your doctors whether to put a cold compress in it or not. The most common thing to do after surgery is to ice it. It helps to reduce the pain, stops it from swelling and bruising.
- Take your prescription medicine on time. Your doctor will prescribe you anti-inflammatory drugs. Make sure to take it with food intake and on time.
- Elevate your legs to keep the blood from flowing normally. This technique may take pressure off your veins and allow them to heal faster.
- Wear your compression stocking. It can help you to recover faster. Wear it for at least two weeks after your surgery.
- Do not drive or travel for at least two weeks. Be patient, it usually takes a year to recover, but it is wiser to talk to your doctor.

Conclusion

Having varicose veins is very discomforting. Most women find it very unappealing. We cannot wear shorts, skirts or sexy dresses without wearing any stockings. I mainly have long legs. It is one of my best assets, but I cannot flaunt them.

Most of us who experience varicose veins have so many concerns, dilemmas and most importantly it causes us a lot of common stress.

Some cannot function well because they keep on thinking about it.

Middle-aged women predominantly suffer from this, and the more you age, the more it is a risk of having or developing varicose veins. We bore children, had hormonal imbalances, worked a long shift, had a very unhealthy diet, and our lifestyles worsened as we aged. Some didn't notice it until they could feel pain and could see traces of it. Some notice it but ignore it until they realize it's too late for them.

It's like it is a little bit too late for us to realize that all those we enjoy, like high heels and high salt foods, are the reasons for our dilemma now. It may be sad, but we have to think that it is not the end of everything.

In a modern world, now we have many ways to prevent and cure varicose veins. Most of them are very easy to reach and acquire. You just look it up on the internet or purchase it in a Pharmacy but the smarter way is to ask your doctor or ask for professional help.

Modern sciences introduce products and cosmetics to hide and ease our problems. All we have to do is to be mindful and resourceful. Doctors now even teach non-surgical ways to cure them. As long as we have faith and determination, we can help ourselves get back on track even though we have it. We have to have discipline in ourselves and eagerness to follow what our doctors say.

I am so glad I followed my friend's advice seeing that kind and good Doctor. He prescribed me a trial bottle of "Venorex. " An all-natural ingredient botanical cream for varicose and thread veins on the legs. It is so unique because it has herbal extracts and other clinically proven ingredients.

Honestly, I am a person who doesn't have time to surf the internet. I am not the kind who usually just trusts products that I am not familiar with and mostly these products are featured or advertised online. Although there are also products that are available in the department store, I am a typical mother who stays in the grocery areas most of the time.

The product contains highly concentrated botanical extracts, anti-aging peptides, vitamins, and other specially selected ingredients that have been combined to help reduce the appearance of varicose veins, spider and thread veins on the skin and legs. It is so safe to use.

The best thing is that it comes with a program based on an eBook. It will teach you the best exercise and diet that will help you decrease or lessen the appearance of your varicose veins.

If you follow the program, it will be life-changing for you too. And one other thing, you can buy it in stores anywhere, it is like it is your reach.

It is an alternative to laser and other surgical treatments.

From my own experience after applying them to my legs, I've

noticed that it improves my skin tone as well. After three weeks of using them religiously, I have seen improvements, and the traces look good.

It's a life-changing situation because I thought my case was the worst, and I never thought it would be corrected, and it would be this easy. I am preparing myself for the worst, like surgery and all, because I wanted to live my life without worries and discomfort.

I just had my love life back, to be like and like before, with Jason, my world was a little bit lighter again, I finally had got my strength back, it's like I am looking forward to going to work with a smile on my face.

Having my kids means the world to me, but this blooming relationship with Jason is an overwhelming feeling I cannot ignore. I am singing in the shower again and feeling young and confident again.

With the help of "Venorex, "I am knocking my way on my mind-blowing dates with Jason. Now I know it will be perfect because I am not bothered with these varicose veins issue, and I will have full attention with my beautiful date, and hopefully, I will get all the kisses that I longed for.

Thank you, "Venorex," You changed my life and gave me hope to be stunning and beautiful again. There is hope with "Venorex" to all the ladies there; never be afraid to ask a doctor or professional help regarding your varicose veins.

Remember, it is never too late for anything. You have to be aware of what is going on in your body. Never let yourself go, always find time and a way to look after yourself. It is not your fault if you developed these kinds of things. It is very natural especially to women who got pregnant or are getting older.

It is very common but most of us do not have a clue how to deal with it. So, because we are not well informed and lack all the information, the next thing we know, it grows bigger or gives us discomfort.

So, before we think that it's too late, we must take action. Always make sure to explore your body and find time to pamper it once in a while. Single mothers like me still have a chance to fall in love again.

Being wanted and loved by a man is the most overwhelming feeling to us. Just like me, I am 48 and Fabulous. Just take my advice, and you can enjoy life and dating without any discomfort and worries. After all, it is never too late to fall in love again.

We were able to get you a trial bottle of Venorex only through the link at https://bit.ly/veno311

www.ingramcontent.com/pod-product-compliance
Lightning Source LLC
Chambersburg PA
CBHW022107020426
42335CB00012B/866